Worker Safety and Health
at Department of Energy Sites

GAO U.S. GOVERNMENT ACCOUNTABILITY OFFICE

441 G St. N.W.
Washington, DC 20548

May 29, 2013

Congressional Committees

Subject: *Worker Safety and Health at Department of Energy Sites*

Work carried out at Department of Energy (DOE) sites across the country involves, among other things, (1) research on dangerous nuclear materials, such as plutonium, and (2) the handling and disposal of radioactive and hazardous waste that, if not handled safely, could cause nuclear accidents or expose the public and the environment to heavy doses of radiation. Workers at DOE sites also perform a wide range of other activities not involving nuclear materials, including construction, routine maintenance, and operating equipment, all of which run the risk of accidents. The consequences of these accidents could be less severe than those involving nuclear materials but could nevertheless result in injuries, long-term illnesses, or even death.

Under the Occupational Safety and Health (OSH) Act of 1970, as amended, the Department of Labor's (Labor) Occupational Safety and Health Administration (OSHA) issues and enforces occupational health and safety regulations. OSHA, or a state with approval from OSHA, regulates the occupational health and safety of private sector employees unless another federal agency has and exercises its statutory authority to regulate. According to the DOE, the Atomic Energy Act (AEA) of 1954, as amended, authorizes DOE to regulate the occupational safety and health of private sector employees at facilities subject to the act. DOE has exercised this authority by issuing various departmental orders, directives, and regulations. In 2006, DOE promulgated regulations—10 C.F.R. Part 851 (Part 851)—which currently govern contractors' worker safety and health at certain DOE sites. DOE relies on contractors and subcontractors to perform day-to-day operations at most of its nuclear and nonnuclear facilities located at approximately 40 sites across the country. In recent years, DOE contractors as well as members of Congress have raised the possibility of revising Part 851 or making a federal agency other than DOE responsible for regulating worker health and safety at the National Nuclear Security Administration (NNSA), a separately organized agency within DOE responsible for the management and security of the nation's nuclear weapons programs.

This report formally transmits the briefing slides presented to committee staff on March 12 and 14, 2013, in response to Senate Report No. 112-173, accompanying S. 3254, a version of the National Defense Authorization Act for Fiscal Year 2013, that directed GAO to review Part 851. The objectives of this report are to identify (1) key similarities and differences between Part 851, OSHA regulations, and the OSH Act; and (2) views of DOE, Labor, and OSHA officials; union representatives; and contractor representatives on whether Part 851 is equally, less, or more protective than OSHA regulations and the OSH Act.

To identify key similarities and differences, we reviewed Part 851, OSHA regulations, the OSH Act, supplemental information for the Part 851 final rule, and a crosswalk document prepared by officials in DOE's Office of Health, Safety, and Security. We also discussed similarities and differences with officials from DOE's Office of Health, Safety, and Security; Office of General Counsel; and NNSA; and Labor's OSHA and Office of the Solicitor. To identify views comparing the protectiveness of Part 851 regulations to OSHA regulations and the OSH Act, we interviewed DOE, Labor, and OSHA officials and reviewed documents, including the National Laboratory Directors Council's (NLDC) analyses of Part 851. We also interviewed representatives from the United Steelworkers and AFL-CIO, which we selected based on our review of relevant literature identifying unions active in the area of Part 851 regulations. In addition, we interviewed contractor representatives at Sandia National Laboratory (SNL). We selected SNL because, among other reasons, NLDC's representative for Part 851 issues and contractor staff who have surveyed contractors at other DOE laboratories about Part 851 work at SNL. Because we selected and interviewed nonprobability samples of union and contractor representatives, their views are not generalizeable to other contractors or union representatives.

We conducted this review from November 2012 to May 2013 in accordance with generally accepted government auditing standards. Those standards require that we plan and perform the audit to obtain sufficient, appropriate evidence to provide a reasonable basis for our findings and conclusions based on our audit objectives. We believe that the evidence obtained provides a reasonable basis for our findings and conclusions based on our audit objectives.

In summary, we found the following:

- There are several key similarities and differences between Part 851, OSHA regulations, and the OSH Act. Several key similarities are that Part 851 incorporates by reference almost all OSHA standards; authorizes workers to file complaints about unsafe working conditions or hazards in the workplace; and requires employers to record occupational fatalities, injuries, and illnesses and retain the records. Several key differences are that Part 851 incorporates additional industry standards and authorizes DOE to accept hazard controls—in certain nonoperational facilities—that are not otherwise fully compliant with applicable DOE regulations for worker health and safety.

- The DOE, Labor, and OSHA officials, and union and contractor representatives we interviewed cited various Part 851 regulations as either equally protective or more protective than OSHA regulations and the OSH Act; only one Part 851 standard was cited as possibly less protective and only by contractor representatives. DOE officials and union and contractor representatives generally viewed Part 851 as at least as protective as OSHA regulations and the OSH Act because it incorporates essentially all OSHA standards and has a general duty clause—which requires employers to protect the health and safety of workers even when no specific standards exist—as does the OSH Act. Contractor representatives viewed one Part 851 standard—an industry standard for respiratory protection—as being less protective than OSHA regulations. However, DOE officials stated that Part 851 also incorporates by reference OSHA's respiratory protection standard and is therefore no less protective. DOE and OSHA officials as well as union and contractor representatives viewed some Part 851 regulations as probably more protective than OSHA regulations. For example, DOE officials and union representatives cited DOE's beryllium standard as being more protective than the OSHA's standard, in part, because DOE's standard has a lower airborne beryllium level that triggers monitoring and protective actions, and DOE officials and contractor representatives cited Part 851's explosive standards as being more applicable to hazards found at DOE sites.

We provided a draft of this report to DOE and OSHA for their review and comment. We received technical comments from both agencies, which we addressed as appropriate.

We are not making any recommendations in this report. See the enclosure for the briefing slides that provide additional details on the results of our review.

- - - - -

We are sending copies of this report to the Secretary of Energy, Secretary of Labor, Assistant Secretary of Labor for Occupational Safety and Health, appropriate congressional committees, and other interested parties. This report also is available at no charge on the GAO website at http://www.gao.gov.

If you or your staff have any questions, please contact me at (202) 512-3841 or trimbled@gao.gov. Contact points for our Offices of Congressional Relations and Public Affairs may be found on the last page of this report. Key contributors to this report were Dan Feehan, Assistant Director; John Delicath; Terry Hanford; Heather Salinas; Jeanette Soares; and Kiki Theodoropoulos.

David C. Trimble
Director, Natural Resources and Environment

Enclosure

List of Committees

The Honorable Carl Levin
Chairman
The Honorable James M. Inhofe
Ranking Member
Committee on Armed Services
United States Senate

The Honorable Dianne Feinstein
Chairman
The Honorable Lamar Alexander
Ranking Member
Subcommittee on Energy and Water Development
Committee on Appropriations
United States Senate

The Honorable Howard P. "Buck" McKeon
Chairman
The Honorable Adam Smith
Ranking Member
Committee on Armed Services
House of Representatives

The Honorable Rodney P. Frelinghuysen
Chairman
The Honorable Marcy Kaptur
Ranking Member
Subcommittee on Energy and Water Development, and Related Agencies
Committee on Appropriations
House of Representatives

Enclosure

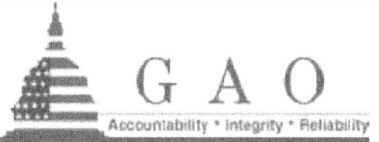

Briefing on Part 851, OSHA Regulations, and the OSH Act

For Congressional Committees

March 2013

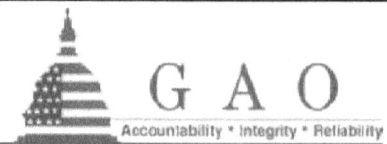

Contents

Page 2

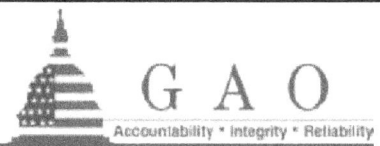

Introduction

- According to the Department of Energy (DOE), the Atomic Energy Act (AEA) of 1954, as amended, authorizes DOE to regulate occupational safety and health of private sector employees at facilities subject to the act. DOE has exercised this authority by issuing various departmental orders, other directives, and regulations.

- Under the Occupational Safety and Health (OSH) Act of 1970, as amended, the Occupational Safety and Health Administration (OSHA) or a state that operates under a plan approved by OSHA, regulates the occupational health and safety of private sector employees unless a federal agency has and exercises statutory authority to regulate those employees. DOE regulates at its sites where it exercises its statutory authority under AEA.

Page 3

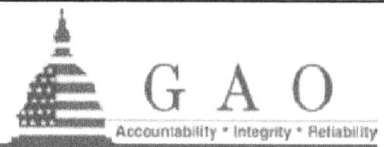

Introduction

- Since the 1990s, various parties have proposed that OSHA, rather than DOE, regulate worker health and safety at DOE sites. In general, the proposals were focused initially on all DOE regulated sites, then focused on DOE science laboratories, and later refocused on the National Nuclear Security Administration (NNSA), a separately organized agency within DOE. (See chronology in app. I.)

- In 2002, the AEA was amended to require DOE to promulgate regulations for industrial and construction health and safety at certain sites. In 2006, DOE promulgated such regulations, specifically 10 C.F.R. Part 851, "Worker Safety and Health Program," which currently governs the conduct of contractor activities at certain DOE sites.

- According to DOE officials, Part 851 programs are one aspect of DOE's Integrated Safety Management System (ISMS), which is designed to ensure that DOE and contractors systematically integrate safety into management and work practices. Under the ISMS, a contractor must define the work to be performed, analyze the potential hazards associated with the work, and identify a set of standards and controls that are sufficient to ensure safety and health if implemented properly.

Page 4

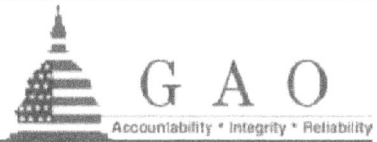

Introduction

- In recent years, DOE contractors and Congress raised the possibility of changes, such as revising Part 851 or changing the agency responsible for regulating worker health and safety at NNSA sites.

- For example, in 2011, the National Laboratory Director Council's (NLDC)—an organization formed by the laboratory directors from each of the 17 DOE national laboratories—prepared a paper on burdensome policies and practices at DOE sites. The paper stated that Part 851—which goes beyond OSHA standards— imposes additional costs without having been shown to increase worker protection. It recommended revising Part 851 to implement only OSHA standards.

Page 5

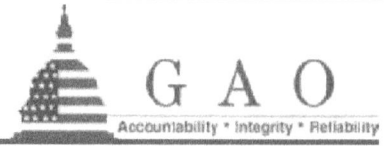

Objectives

Senate Report No. 112-173 accompanying S. 3254, a version of the National Defense Authorization Act for Fiscal Year 2013, requested GAO to review Part 851. In response, our objectives were to identify:

1. key similarities and differences between Part 851, OSHA regulations, and the OSH Act; and

2. views of DOE, Labor, and OSHA officials; union representatives; and contractor representatives on whether the Part 851 regulation is equally, less, or more protective than OSHA regulations and the OSH Act.

Page 6

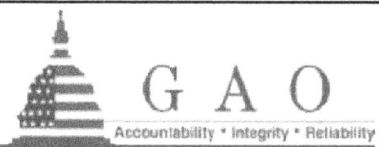

Scope and Methodology

- To identify key similarities and differences, we reviewed Part 851, OSHA regulations, the OSH Act, supplemental information for the Part 851 final rule, and a crosswalk document prepared by officials in DOE's Office of Health, Safety, and Security.

- For both Objectives 1 and 2, we conducted interviews with

    - officials from DOE's Office of Health, Safety, and Security; Office of General Counsel; and NNSA;

    - officials from Department of Labor's OSHA and Office of the Solicitor;

    - contractor representatives for the NLDC and Sandia National Laboratory; and

    - representatives from United Steelworkers and AFL-CIO.

Page 7

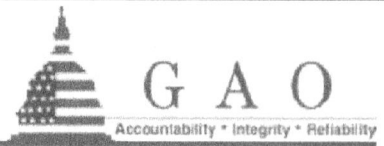

Scope and Methodology

- To identify views comparing the protectiveness of Part 851 regulations to OSHA regulations and the OSH Act, we interviewed DOE, Labor, and OSHA officials and reviewed documents including NLDC's analyses of Part 851.

- We selected representatives from two union organizations to interview, based on our review of relevant literature that indicated these were active unions in the area of Part 851 regulations.

- We selected contractor representatives at Sandia National Laboratory to interview, based on several criteria, including that Sandia National Laboratory is the location of the NLDC representative for Part 851 issues and contractor staff who had surveyed contractors at other DOE laboratories concerning Part 851 issues. Both the union and contractor representatives are nongeneralizable samples.

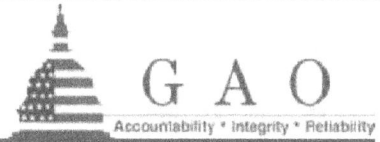

Scope and Methodology

- We obtained technical comments from DOE and OSHA and incorporated those comments as appropriate.

- We conducted this performance audit from November 2012 to mid-March 2013 in accordance with generally accepted government auditing standards. Those standards require that we plan and perform the audit to obtain sufficient appropriate evidence to provide a reasonable basis for our findings and conclusions based on our audit objectives. We believe that the evidence obtained provides a reasonable basis for our findings and conclusions based on our audit objectives.

Page 9

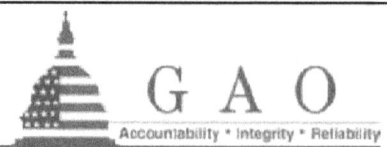

Background

- OSHA issues and enforces occupational safety and health standards for workplaces that are not regulated by other federal agencies. Such standards require conditions, or the adoption or use of practices, means, methods, operations, or processes, reasonably necessary or appropriate to provide safe or healthful employment and places of employment.

- The OSH Act directed the Secretary of Labor to adopt any national consensus standards or established federal standards as safety and health standards within 2 years of the date the OSH Act went into effect in 1971.

- In 2012, we reported that the vast majority of OSHA standards have not changed since first adopted in the 1970s and that it takes an average of more than 7 years for OSHA to develop and issue new safety standards.[1]

[1]GAO, *Workplace Safety and Health: Multiple Challenges Lengthen OSHA's Standard Setting*, GAO-12-330 (Washington, D.C.: Apr. 2, 2012).

Page 10

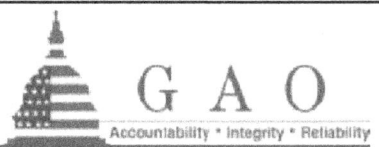

Objective 1: Key Similarities between Part 851 and OSHA Regulations and the OSH Act

- Part 851 is similar to the OSH Act and OSHA regulations by

  - incorporating by reference almost all OSHA standards;

  - requiring employers to protect the health and safety of workers, even when no specific standard exists, a requirement known as the general duty clause;

  - authorizing workers to file complaints about unsafe working conditions or hazards in the workplace; and

  - establishing processes to inspect workplaces and investigate potential violations.

Page 11

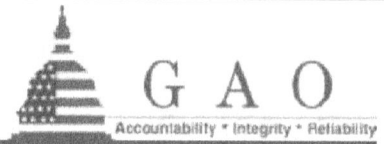

Objective 1: Key Similarities between Part 851and OSHA Regulations and the OSH Act

- Part 851 is similar to the OSH Act and OSHA regulations by (continued)

    - establishing enforcement processes after investigating potential violations; and

    - requiring employers to record occupational fatalities, injuries, and illnesses and retain the records.

Page 12

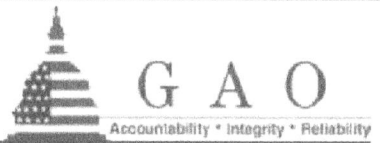

Objective 1: Key Differences between Part 851and OSHA Regulations and the OSH Act

- Part 851 differs from OSHA regulations and the OSH Act by

  - authorizing DOE to issue compliance orders—which, among other things, can mandate a work stoppage or action to remedy a hazard. According to OSHA officials, the agency would have to obtain a court order to force an employer to stop work because of an imminent danger, although employers often will stop work if OSHA notifies them of an imminent danger.

  - authorizing DOE to assess different types and amounts of penalties.

Page 13

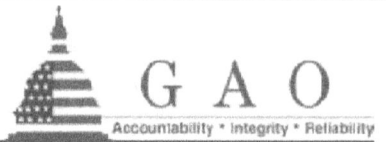

Objective 1: Key Differences between Part 851and OSHA Regulations

- Part 851 differs from OSHA regulations by (continued)

  - including standards for certain hazards, such as beryllium, that contain different requirements than OSHA standards;

  - including standards that cover hazards not covered by OSHA standards, such as firearms safety; and

  - incorporating a more current version of industry standards and guidelines (e.g., voluntary industry consensus standards).

Page 14

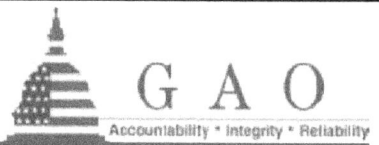

Objective 1: Key Differences between Part 851and OSHA Regulations

- Part 851 differs from OSHA regulations by (continued)

    - requiring contractors to prepare a written worker safety and health program that addresses all Part 851 requirements and applicable functional areas, whereas OSHA regulations generally do not require such programs.

    - requiring contractors to establish procedures to permit workers to decline work in certain hazardous conditions, whereas OSHA regulations do not require employers to establish such procedures, but the regulations also permit workers to decline work in certain circumstances.

    - requiring contractors to investigate certain accidents, injuries, and illnesses and analyze related data for trends and lessons learned, whereas OSHA regulations do not impose such requirements on employers.

Page 15

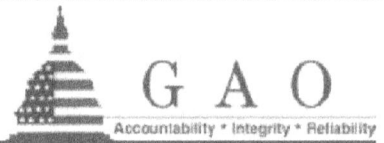

Objective 1: Key Differences between Part 851and OSHA Regulations

- Part 851 differs from OSHA regulations by (continued)

  - requiring contractors to involve workers in (1) developing worker safety and health program goals, objectives and performance measures and (2) identifying and controlling workplace hazards. OSHA regulations do not have a generic requirement for such worker participation; however, specific standards may, and non-mandatory guidance identifies worker involvement in such activities as a best practice;

  - establishing an application procedure for variances from standards overseen by agency officials with whom employees can request a conference, whereas under OSHA regulations, employees can request a variance application hearing, which will be heard by an administrative law judge;

  - requires reporting of all workplace accidents, illness, and injuries to DOE, but OSHA regulations require the reporting of certain incidents;

  - authorizing DOE to accept hazard controls in certain nonoperational facilities that are not otherwise fully compliant with applicable regulations for worker health and safety, whereas OSHA regulations do not.

Page 16

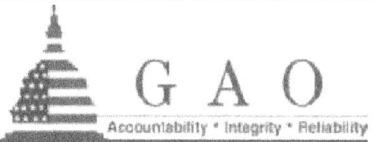

Objective 2: Views on Whether Part 851 Is Equally, Less, or More Protective

- DOE, Labor, and OSHA officials and the union and contractor representatives we interviewed had sometimes divergent views on whether Part 851 regulations are equally, less, or more protective than OSHA regulations and the OSH Act.[2]

[2]Because this information is derived from interviews of a nonprobability sample of contractor and union representatives, the views we present for these representatives are their views only and are not generalizeable to other contractors and union representatives.

Page 17

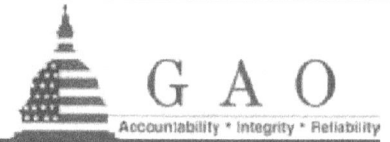

Objective 2: Views on Whether Part 851 Is Equally, Less, or More Protective

Part 851 Regulations Considered <u>Equally</u> Protective:

*   **DOE officials and union and contractor representatives agreed that Part 851 is at least as protective because it incorporates essentially all OSHA standards and has a general duty clause, as does the OSH Act.**

Page 18

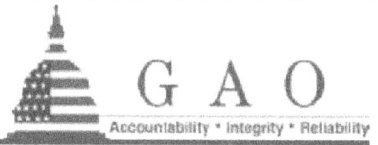

Objective 2: Views on Whether Part 851 Is Equally, Less, or More Protective

Part 851 Regulations Considered <u>Less</u> Protective:

- Part 851 includes an industry standard for respiratory protection, which contractor representatives cited as being less protective than OSHA's respiratory protection standard. In contrast, DOE officials noted that because Part 851 also incorporates by reference OSHA's respiratory protection standard, Part 851 cannot be less protective.

Page 19

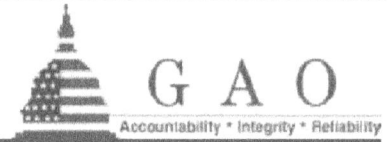

Objective 2: Views on Whether Part 851 Is Equally, Less, or More Protective

Part 851 Regulations Considered <u>More</u> Protective:

*   DOE and OSHA officials as well as union and contractor representatives agreed that at least some Part 851 regulations are probably more protective than OSHA regulations. However, DOE officials, union representatives, and contractor representatives sometimes disagreed on which Part 851 regulations are more protective.

    *   *Beryllium Standard.* According to DOE officials and union representatives, Part 851 is more protective because it has an enhanced standard for beryllium, including a lower airborne beryllium level that triggers monitoring and protective actions. OSHA recognizes that its exposure limit may not provide adequate worker protection.[3]

[3]According to OSHA officials, OSHA is currently developing a proposed standard for beryllium.

Page 20

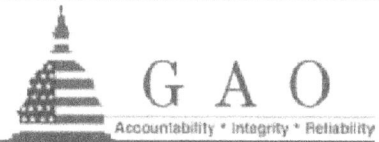

Objective 2: Views on Whether Part 851 Is Equally, Less, or More Protective

Part 851 Regulations Considered <u>More</u> Protective: (continued)

- DOE officials and union representatives stated other industry standards in Part 851 are more up to date than OSHA standards (e.g., air exposure limits for chemicals). However, Labor officials said the general duty clause of the OSH Act might require compliance with more current industry standards, but also acknowledged that it is difficult to prevail in an employer's challenge to enforcement actions brought under the clause.

- DOE officials and contractor representatives stated the electrical standards in Part 851 are more up to date and protective.

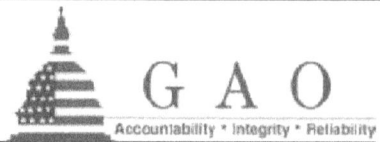

Objective 2: Views on Whether Part 851 Is Equally, Less, or More Protective

Part 851 Regulations Considered <u>More</u> Protective: (continued)

- OSHA regulations do not address certain hazards at DOE sites, which are addressed in Part 851.

    - *Explosives.* DOE officials and contractor representatives said that Part 851's explosive safety standards are more protective than OSHA standards because OSHA does not have explosive safety standards specific to nuclear environments, which exist at DOE sites.

    - *Firearms.* DOE and OSHA officials said that Part 851 has safety standards for firearms as used at DOE sites but that OSHA does not have comparable standards.

    - *Lasers.* DOE officials and contractor representatives said that Part 851's laser safety standard is more protective because relevant OSHA standards only apply to construction activities, which would not cover all laser operations at DOE sites. However, OSHA officials said that, although OSHA does not have an industry standard specifically for lasers, other OSHA standards—such as eye protection standards—would protect workers from injurious light.

Page 22

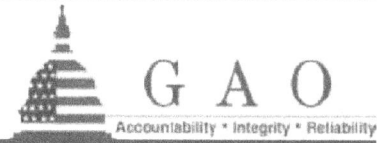

Objective 2: Views on Whether Part 851 Is Equally, Less, or More Protective

Part 851 Regulations Considered <u>More</u> Protective:

- OSHA regulations generally do not require employers to establish certain safety and health programs, which are addressed in Part 851.

  - *Worker Safety and Health Program.* DOE officials and union representatives said such programs enhance protectiveness by ensuring proactive and comprehensive attention to hazards at DOE sites. According to one DOL official, OSHA encourages employers to develop such programs but does not require them, except in the area of construction.

  - *Functional Areas.* DOE officials and union representatives said that to ensure attention to common DOE site hazards, Part 851 requires health and safety programs tailored to 10 specific areas, such as industrial hygiene and firearms safety. OSHA officials said similar OSHA regulations are limited to only certain substances, hazards, or standards. Contractor representatives noted, however, that Part 851 regulations for some of these 10 areas are mostly duplicated by OSHA standards and only equally protective.

Page 23

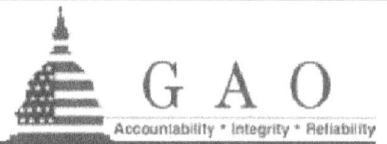

Appendix I: Chronology Illustrating External Regulation Proposals

Since the early 1990s, DOE and others have examined or proposed transitioning from DOE's self-regulation to external regulation by OSHA.

(1993 – 2000)

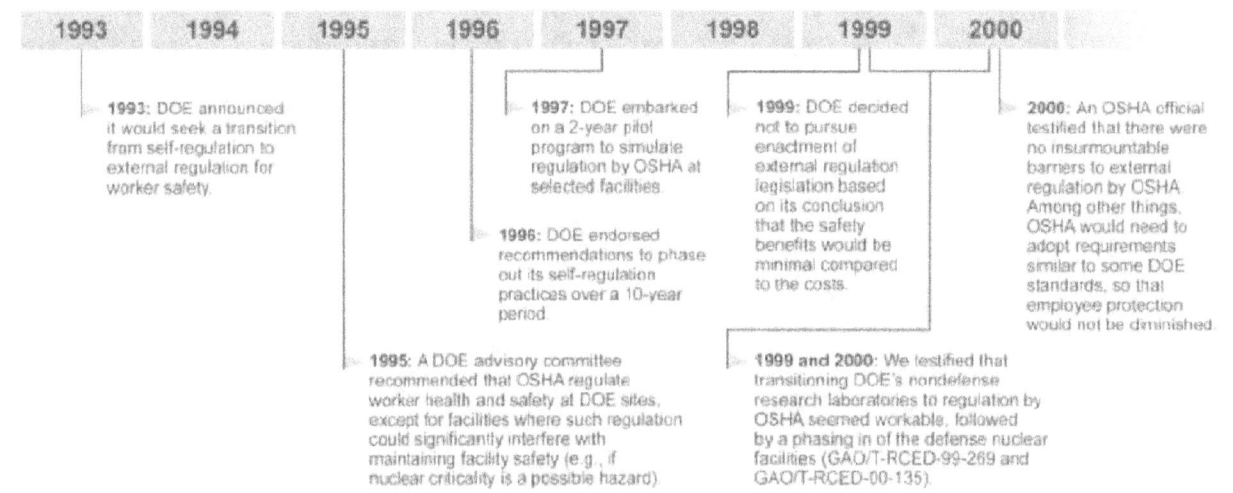

1993: DOE announced it would seek a transition from self-regulation to external regulation for worker safety.

1997: DOE embarked on a 2-year pilot program to simulate regulation by OSHA at selected facilities.

1996: DOE endorsed recommendations to phase out its self-regulation practices over a 10-year period.

1995: A DOE advisory committee recommended that OSHA regulate worker health and safety at DOE sites, except for facilities where such regulation could significantly interfere with maintaining facility safety (e.g., if nuclear criticality is a possible hazard).

1999: DOE decided not to pursue enactment of external regulation legislation based on its conclusion that the safety benefits would be minimal compared to the costs.

2000: An OSHA official testified that there were no insurmountable barriers to external regulation by OSHA. Among other things, OSHA would need to adopt requirements similar to some DOE standards, so that employee protection would not be diminished.

1999 and 2000: We testified that transitioning DOE's nondefense research laboratories to regulation by OSHA seemed workable, followed by a phasing in of the defense nuclear facilities (GAO/T-RCED-99-269 and GAO/T-RCED-00-135).

Page 24

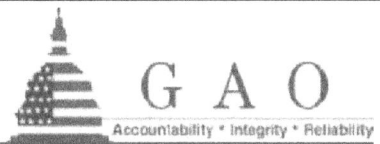

Appendix I: Chronology Illustrating External Regulation Proposals

(2001 – 2012)

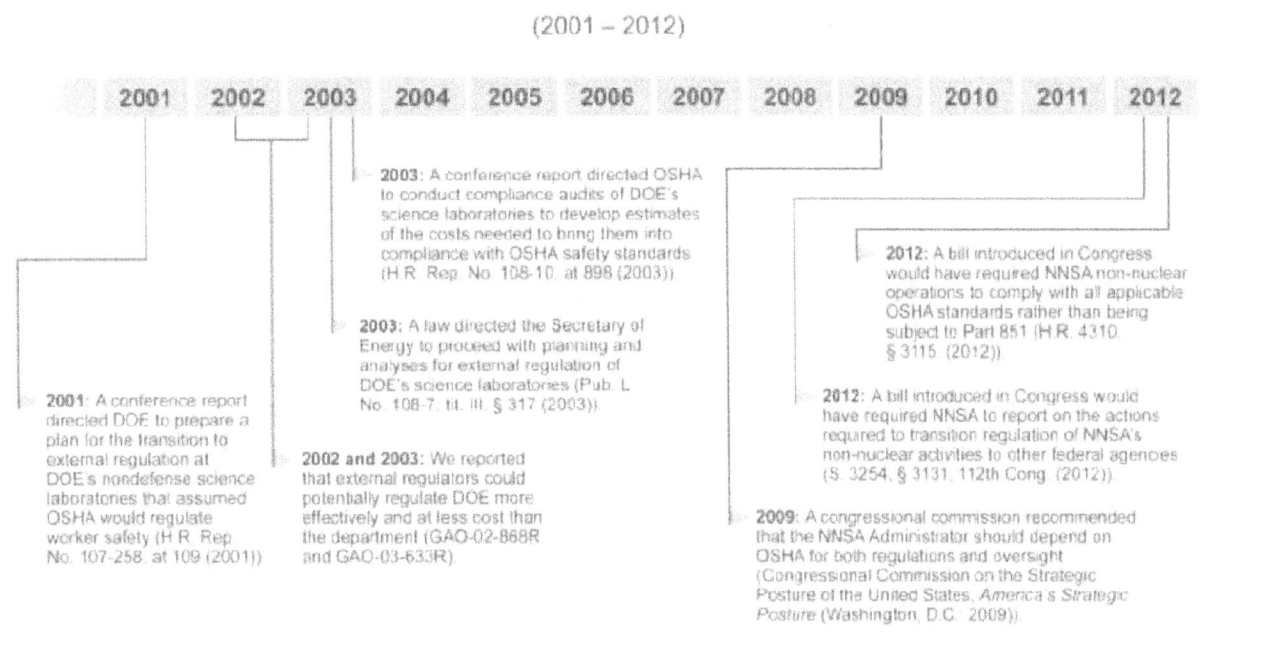

| 2001 | 2002 | 2003 | 2004 | 2005 | 2006 | 2007 | 2008 | 2009 | 2010 | 2011 | 2012 |

2003: A conference report directed OSHA to conduct compliance audits of DOE's science laboratories to develop estimates of the costs needed to bring them into compliance with OSHA safety standards (H.R. Rep. No. 108-10, at 898 (2003)).

2003: A law directed the Secretary of Energy to proceed with planning and analyses for external regulation of DOE's science laboratories (Pub. L. No. 108-7, tit. III, § 317 (2003)).

2001: A conference report directed DOE to prepare a plan for the transition to external regulation at DOE's nondefense science laboratories that assumed OSHA would regulate worker safety (H.R. Rep. No. 107-258, at 109 (2001)).

2002 and 2003: We reported that external regulators could potentially regulate DOE more effectively and at less cost than the department (GAO-02-868R and GAO-03-633R).

2012: A bill introduced in Congress would have required NNSA non-nuclear operations to comply with all applicable OSHA standards rather than being subject to Part 851 (H.R. 4310, § 3115. (2012)).

2012: A bill introduced in Congress would have required NNSA to report on the actions required to transition regulation of NNSA's non-nuclear activities to other federal agencies (S. 3254, § 3131, 112th Cong. (2012)).

2009: A congressional commission recommended that the NNSA Administrator should depend on OSHA for both regulations and oversight (Congressional Commission on the Strategic Posture of the United States, *America's Strategic Posture* (Washington, D.C. 2009)).

Page 25

(361456)

GAO's Mission	The Government Accountability Office, the audit, evaluation, and investigative arm of Congress, exists to support Congress in meeting its constitutional responsibilities and to help improve the performance and accountability of the federal government for the American people. GAO examines the use of public funds; evaluates federal programs and policies; and provides analyses, recommendations, and other assistance to help Congress make informed oversight, policy, and funding decisions. GAO's commitment to good government is reflected in its core values of accountability, integrity, and reliability.
Obtaining Copies of GAO Reports and Testimony	The fastest and easiest way to obtain copies of GAO documents at no cost is through GAO's website (www.gao.gov). Each weekday afternoon, GAO posts on its website newly released reports, testimony, and correspondence. To have GAO e-mail you a list of newly posted products, go to www.gao.gov and select "E-mail Updates."
Order by Phone	The price of each GAO publication reflects GAO's actual cost of production and distribution and depends on the number of pages in the publication and whether the publication is printed in color or black and white. Pricing and ordering information is posted on GAO's website, http://www.gao.gov/ordering.htm. Place orders by calling (202) 512-6000, toll free (866) 801-7077, or TDD (202) 512-2537. Orders may be paid for using American Express, Discover Card, MasterCard, Visa, check, or money order. Call for additional information.
Connect with GAO	Connect with GAO on Facebook, Flickr, Twitter, and YouTube. Subscribe to our RSS Feeds or E-mail Updates. Listen to our Podcasts. Visit GAO on the web at www.gao.gov.
To Report Fraud, Waste, and Abuse in Federal Programs	Contact: Website: www.gao.gov/fraudnet/fraudnet.htm E-mail: fraudnet@gao.gov Automated answering system: (800) 424-5454 or (202) 512-7470
Congressional Relations	Katherine Siggerud, Managing Director, siggerudk@gao.gov, (202) 512-4400, U.S. Government Accountability Office, 441 G Street NW, Room 7125, Washington, DC 20548
Public Affairs	Chuck Young, Managing Director, youngc1@gao.gov, (202) 512-4800 U.S. Government Accountability Office, 441 G Street NW, Room 7149 Washington, DC 20548

www.ingramcontent.com/pod-product-compliance
Lightning Source LLC
Chambersburg PA
CBHW081139280526

45787CB00007B/3156